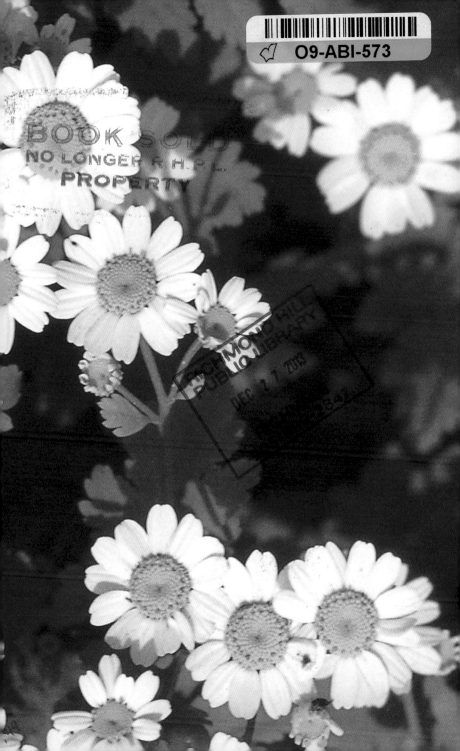

O9-ABI-573

# **50** TIPS TO CURE A
# HEADACHE

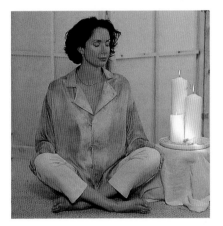

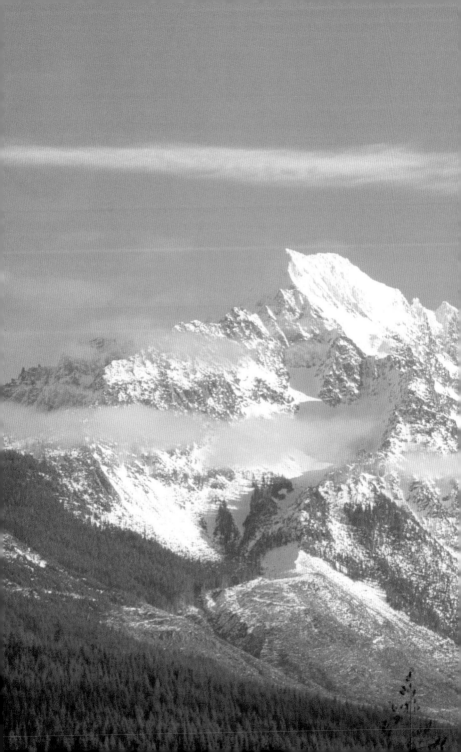

# **50** TIPS TO CURE A
# HEADACHE

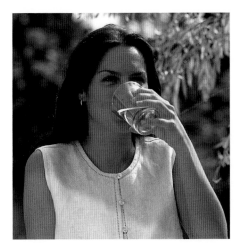

Natural ways to activate the
body's own healing process

Raje Airey

LORENZ BOOKS

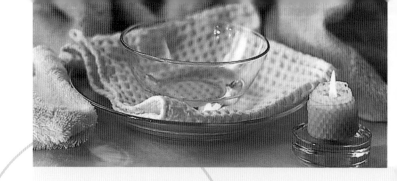

# contents

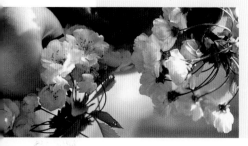

# **50** TIPS TO CURE A
# HEADACHE

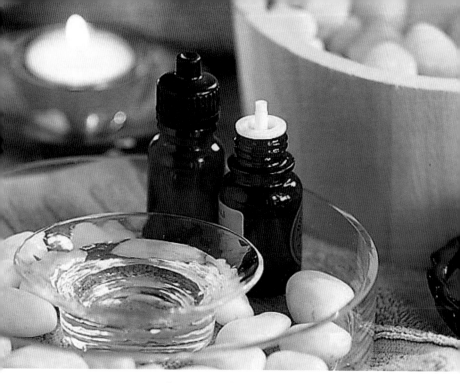

# introduction

Almost everyone knows what it is like to have a headache. It is thought that more than 90 per cent of the population will have experienced a headache at one time or another, and unfortunately for many people they are almost a routine part of life.

There are hundreds of different causes of headaches, both psychological and physiological, and many different types of headache, ranging in severity from a crippling migraine which may last several days to a hangover headache which can clear up in a few hours. In some cases, headaches may indicate a major disorder such as a brain tumour or a life-threatening illness such as meningitis, but this is extremely rare.

Most headaches seen by the family doctor are known as "benign recurring headaches"; the vast majority of these are described as "tension headaches".

### muscle restriction

Tension headaches are so-called because they are usually caused by some type of physical tension in the muscles of the shoulders, neck and head, and by constriction or congestion of the blood vessels in the head. The pain typically arises from the base of the skull (occiput) and extends up over the back of the head to the forehead and temples. The pain results from the continuous, partial contraction of muscles attached to the scalp and can affect the whole head.

◄ *Use essential oil to help relieve a headache. Put a few drops in your bath water, on a handkerchief, or use an aromatherapy oil burner.*

Some people wake up with a headache, which then lasts all day with varying degrees of severity, ranging from a general dull ache to sudden jabbing pains in a particular spot. Other people experience this type of headache as a feeling of pressure, like a tight band around the head, or as a persistent throbbing. Although tension headaches are not associated with visual disturbance, many sufferers dislike bright light and find it hard to concentrate.

## migraines

Many regular headache sufferers describe their condition as "having a migraine". However, a migraine is a specific medical condition and is not the same as an everyday tension headache. Migraines are a fairly common neurological disorder, with three times as many women as men suffering. Many women's migraines occur premenstrually and are linked to hormonal imbalances.

The severe pain of a migraine headache is thought to be caused by the dilation (swelling up) of the blood vessels in the head, causing a disturbance in the flow of blood to the brain. This follows a brief period of constriction of the vessels which partly

▶ *If you have a busy lifestyle, just a few minutes spent meditating each day will reduce the number of headaches you have.*

accounts for the visual disturbances (known as "aura") that many people experience prior to the headache. Migraines cause chemical changes in the body and typical symptoms include aversion to light (photophobia), nausea, vomiting and diarrhoea. The headache itself is often one-sided and is marked by severe pain in the forehead or temples, or rising up from the back of the neck. A migraine attack can last up to 72 hours and becomes extremely debilitating. It can take a day or two after an attack to get back to normal.

## bouts of pain

Cluster headaches are often confused with migraine as the severe pain tends to be centred around the eye area and is typically one-sided. These headaches occur in bouts during a 1–2 month period. In an attack, the headache will come on suddenly and

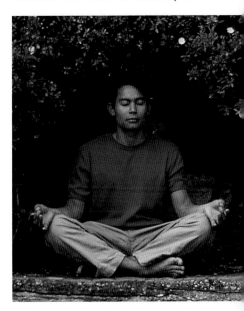

last up to an hour. Several attacks may be experienced in a day, often waking the sufferer from sleep, or causing them to pace about as the pain is so intense. Cluster headaches are less common than migraines; they rarely occur in anyone under 30 and most sufferers are men. Drinking alcohol during a bout can bring on an attack.

### a symptom of another illness

Other types of headache arise as secondary symptoms of problems elsewhere in the body. This may include mechanical injuries, such as whiplash or head injuries, or general wear and tear on the body, caused by failing eyesight, poor posture, or arthritis in the neck, for instance. Similarly, headaches associated with premenstrual syndrome (PMS), high blood pressure, blocked sinuses, inflammation of the middle ear and viral infections are also fairly common.

### headache triggers

Most headaches do not come out of the blue, but are triggered by certain factors. Migraines, cluster and tension headaches are typically linked to stress, overwork and negative emotional states such as worry, anxiety, depression and held-in anger and resentment. After stress, food allergies and/or intolerances are one of the most common causes of migraine and tension headaches. Certain foods, such as red wine, cheese and chocolate, are well-known triggers. Others include low blood sugar, caffeine withdrawal,

lack of sleep and toxicity in the body, caused by poor digestion or over-indulgence in sugar and alcohol, for instance. Long-distance driving, too much sun, changes in the weather and sensitivities to environmental triggers, such as perfume, car exhaust fumes, cigarette smoke and paint fumes, can also play a part.

### nature's remedies

Conventional treatment for a headache is standard painkillers, either available on prescription for migraine and severe headaches, or over-the-counter for everyday tension headaches. The drugs often combine painkillers, such as aspirin or paracetamol, with other drugs which have a sedative, antispasmodic action. Because these drugs are so common and easily available, we tend to think they are harmless and that we can take them every day. While these drugs have their place, they also have many potentially harmful side effects, particularly if taken on a regular basis. It is believed that many people are addicted to painkillers, and that many headaches are caused as the result of taking too many pills. For this reason, increasing numbers of people are turning to natural medicine as they look for effective treatments which are non-habit forming and non-toxic.

This book contains information and ideas for how to treat headaches without using drugs. In natural medicine, pain is seen as the body's way of telling you that something is

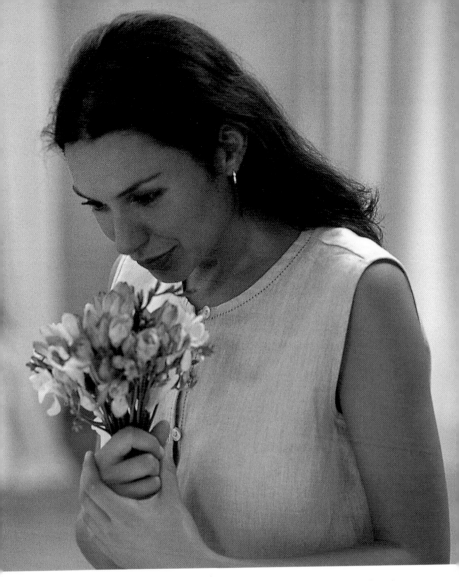

wrong; it has a protective function, acting as an "early warning system". Consequently, many of the treatments are based on dealing with the underlying cause of the pain and recognizing the importance of diet, lifestyle and psychological factors. Natural remedies can be used to help

▲ *Most people appreciate the soft and subtle scent of flowers. Their gentle perfume can help relieve a headache.*

the body work through its own healing process with minimum discomfort. Use it as a guide to find a treatment that is just right for you.

# headache
# treatments

The treatments in this book are based on holistic principles. This means they have an underlying assumption that good health depends on a balance between physical, mental, emotional and spiritual wellbeing. The treatments are drawn from a wide variety of natural-healing traditions; some of these practices have been used for centuries as an aid to health and wellbeing. They are all based on therapeutic techniques which help to stimulate the body's own natural healing ability, and include hands-on therapies such as massage, shiatsu and reflexology as well as treatments based on herbal remedies, aromatherapy and nutrition. There are also treatments to relieve stress and tension, such as meditation and yoga, and subtle energy healing methods using reiki, crystals and colour.

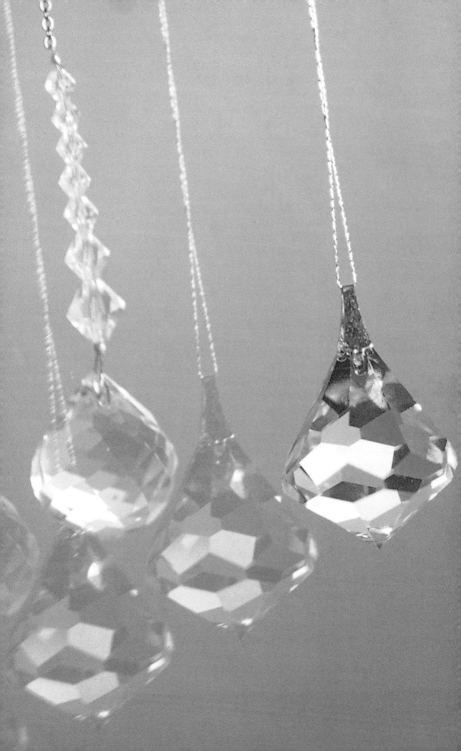

# 1

# refreshing water

The body of a healthy adult is made up of about 75 per cent water. Water is vital for life, yet many common health problems, such as headaches, are linked with dehydration.

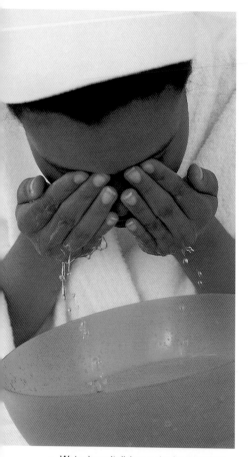

▲ *Water is revitalizing and refreshing and an excellent panacea for a headache.*

Start the day with a glass of water. This flushes out your kidneys and detoxifies your system. Water is best drunk half an hour before eating and between meals, to allow for the flushing action and to avoid interfering with the body's digestive processes.

At the first sign of a headache, drink a couple of glasses of water. Often this is enough for it to lift without the need for further treatment. Add a slice of lemon for a refreshing tang and a burst of vitamin C to kick-start the liver. Drinking water when stressed or anxious also helps to keep your body fluids flowing smoothly and can help to calm you down.

To dispel headaches brought on by eyestrain, try splashing the eyes and forehead with warm and then cold water. This stimulates the circulation and refreshes tired eyes.

**KEEP HYDRATED**
Alcohol, tea, coffee and fizzy drinks are diuretics; for every drink it is recommended to drink at least one glass of water to counter its effect.

# 2 regular exercise

Exercise is one of the best stress-busting methods around. During exercise, the body burns off excess adrenalin, so if you suffer from tension headaches, make exercise an everyday part of life.

When we are stressed, the body responds by producing extra adrenalin as its "fight or flight" mechanism comes into force. If this adrenalin is not used, it overloads the system and gets stored in the body, creating tense, tight muscles, which leads to headaches. No matter what your age, weight or physical build, there will be some form of exercise that is right for you.

**keep focused**

One of the hardest things about exercise is staying motivated. Enthusiasm may be high at the beginning of a new regime, but typically wanes as the weeks go by.

Most importantly, first find a method of exercise that you like: if you don't like it, you won't do it. This could be running, yoga, swimming, walking, gardening, t'ai chi, playing a team sport or joining the gym. Then build exercise into your normal routine so that it becomes as much of an everyday activity as eating or washing.

If you are very busy, find opportunities for exercise in regular activities: take the stairs instead of the elevator; cycle or walk rather than use the car; or use a manual lawnmower to mow the grass. If exercise doesn't come naturally, remember that it can be fun as well as beneficial.

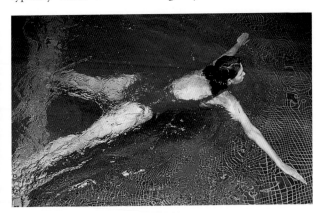

◀ Swimming is a good all-round exercise to do. The water supports your body so the exercise remains gentle and won't add to your headache.

# 3 easy neck stretches

Many tension headaches begin with a feeling of pressure in the head or at the base of the neck. A few simple stretches can help to relieve this muscular tension before the headache kicks in.

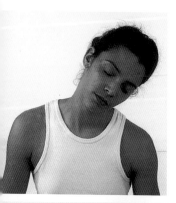

**head and neck stretch**
**1** Turn the head to one side, then slowly rotate it in a semicircular movement, letting the chin drop down across the chest. Repeat in the opposite direction.

**2** For an extra stretch, slowly stretch your head down to one side, feeling the pull in the neck muscles. Use your hands as a lever to make this side stretch more effective. Place one hand under your chin and the other on top of your head; as you stretch sideways, exert a steady pressure with both hands, but be careful not to pull or tug your head. Change hands and repeat on the other side.

**face work-out**

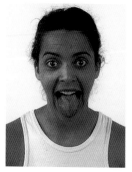

Another area where you hold a lot of tension is the face. This simple exercise is excellent for stretching the delicate facial muscles to release tension. To do it, find a quiet spot where you are unobserved. Open your mouth as wide as possible and push out your tongue. At the same time, open your eyes into as wide a stare as you can manage. Hold for a moment or two then relax. Repeat a couple of times.

4

# relaxing yoga positions

Yoga relaxes the muscles, slows the breath and brings stillness to the mind, making it a useful therapy for treating stress-related disorders. These two poses can be undertaken by anyone.

**standing bend (right)**
Place a headrest on a stool. Stand with your feet parallel and hip width apart. Breathe out and bend forwards from the hips slowly. Rest your arms over your head on the stool and relax for 1–2 minutes.

**lying flat (below)**
Lie on a flat surface, with your legs and arms releasing out to the sides. Use a cushion if you feel more comfortable. Close your eyes and relax for 10–15 minutes.

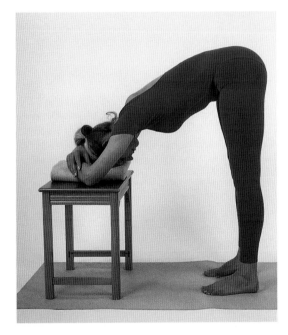

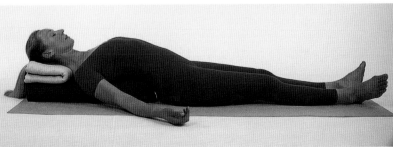

# 5 healthy eating

Food fuels the body. Frequent headaches may be linked to a poor diet, so it is worth spending time preparing meals from good quality, fresh ingredients rather than using convenience foods.

A well-balanced diet is rich in fibre, vitamins and minerals; this means eating plenty of fresh fruit and vegetables, wholegrains such as rice, millet and barley, and wholegrain bread and cereals. For protein, eat a little lean meat, poultry, fish, cheese, nuts and soya products.

## B-complex vitamins

Having enough of the B-complex vitamins is necessary for the healthy functioning of the nervous system. They get used up more rapidly when we are under stress. Studies have shown that niacin ($B_3$) can help prevent and ease the severity of migraines. The best natural sources are in liver, kidney, lean meat, wholegrains, brewer's yeast, wheat germ, fish, eggs, roasted peanuts, the white meat of poultry, avocados, dates, figs and prunes.

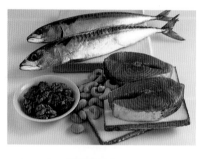

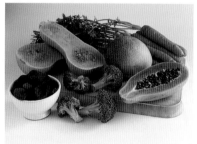

▲ *Choose organic products as these are free from potentially harmful toxic residues.*

### HEALTHY CHOICES
If you are prone to headaches, cut down on your intake of processed foods, sugar, salt, refined carbohydrates, tea, coffee, fizzy drinks and alcohol.

Many common foods contain chemicals that can trigger neural and blood vessel changes in the brain, causing migraines or severe headaches in susceptible people. Common migraine triggers are chocolate, citrus fruits, cheese, coffee, bacon and alcohol, particularly red wine.

# 6 quick-fix snacks

Many headaches are caused by a low blood-sugar level. As your energy level drops, don't be tempted to go for an instant fix with caffeine or sugar, instead choose healthy snacks.

There are many steps you can take to help break an unhealthy cycle. Avoid the temptation to snack unhealthily or to miss meals and "eat on the run". A few nuts or seeds or a piece of fresh fruit is a good substitute for a chocolate bar or bag of crisps (potato chips).

## healthy food rules

Eating little and often is a good habit to cultivate. Eat regular light meals, based on fresh, whole ingredients, every

▼ *Complex carbohydrates are the best source of energy. Nuts are filling and release energy slowly.*

3–4 hours. This will help to stabilize your blood sugar level and prevent excessive energy swings. You should feel better and notice an improvement in your headaches.

Monitor your intake of caffeinated drinks and limit yourself to no more than one or two cups of tea or coffee a day. There are many replacements, such as herbal teas and cereal coffees made from barley, rye, chicory or acorns for instance, which are available in good health stores. Replace sugar with a little fructose (fruit sugar) or honey, either of which is preferable to an artificial sweetener or refined sugar.

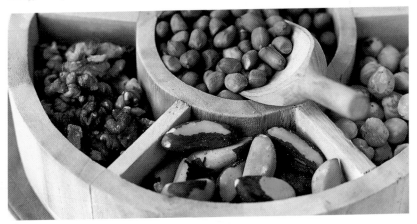

# 7 identifying food intolerance

Most migraine sufferers are aware that certain foods and drinks can trigger an attack. Frequent headaches may also be a symptom of widespread and recognized food allergies or intolerances.

Food intolerance is when the body becomes hypersensitive to certain foods; the immune system perceives the substance as harmful, and sets off a chain reaction in the body which produces various symptoms, including sneezing, itchy rashes, sinus problems, lethargy, an uncomfortable bloated feeling and headaches. The onset of food intolerance can occur at any age and to a substance that was previously tolerated. The only way of finding out if you have a food intolerance is to eliminate the suspect food/s from your diet, one at a time, and see whether your symptoms disappear. Common

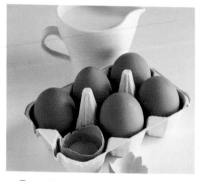

▲ Try cutting out cow's milk or eggs to help your headache symptoms.

offenders include products made from cow's milk, wheat, corn, yeast, eggs, nuts and shellfish.

### plan ahead

If you think you may have a food intolerance and want to try an elimination diet, make sure you plan ahead so that you don't run out of suitable foods. Base your diet on fresh foods and do not skip meals. Avoid eating out, or if you do, choose plainly cooked dishes. Always check the labels on any manufactured foods, in case they contain the foods that you want to eliminate.

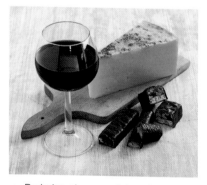

▲ Red wine, cheese and chocolate can bring on migraines for some people.

# 8 green leaf cleanser

Toxicity in the body is one of the principal causes of headaches. Often this is the result of digestive problems such as constipation and/or the absorption of incompletely digested foods.

A sedentary lifestyle combined with a diet low in fibre and water and high in processed foods and caffeinated drinks makes constipation a common health problem. Additionally, regular use of antibiotics and other drugs, alcohol and/or a high intake of sugar can lead to inflammation of the walls of the small intestine, causing intestinal permeability or a "leaky gut". This means that toxic waste is reabsorbed through the intestinal wall back into the bloodstream, causing headaches, fatigue, skin problems and bad breath.

To improve digestion, increase your daily intake of fibre-rich foods, such as raw fruit and vegetables, brown rice and wholegrains. You should also increase your fluid intake. Filtered water is a must, but for a detox include fresh green vegetable juices.

## green juice

All fresh juices have a cleansing effect on the digestive system and are gently laxative. Celery juice is effective against headaches, and combines well with dark green vegetables (such as kale, watercress and spinach) which are rich in B vitamins and minerals. To make

enough for one serving, you will need 6 large spinach leaves, 2 sticks of celery, plus 2 or 3 tomatoes for flavour. Wash the ingredients and put them through a juice extractor. Serve immediately as fresh juices lose their potency if they are left. If you prefer, you may dilute the juice with water. Drink up to three glasses a day between meals.

▾ Fresh vegetable juices help the body to detoxify and the cells to regenerate and repair themselves.

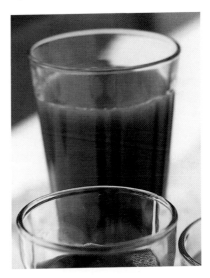

During sex, the body relaxes, easing muscular tension and dissolving energy blocks, which are often the source of headaches. It is one of the best natural therapies there is.

# 10 get a good night's rest

Sleep is one of nature's great healers. During sleep the cells of the body renew and repair themselves. Sleep deprivation can lead to all kinds of physical and emotional problems including headaches.

Sleeplessness is a common response to stress as your mind and body cannot let go enough to give you the rest you need. If you have headaches caused by stress, learning to switch off and relax is essential for promoting restful sleep. Make sure you have a healthy diet, take regular exercise and have a calming routine to wind down before bedtime.

## SLEEP DO'S AND DON'TS

- Get plenty of fresh air and exercise on a regular basis.
- Don't sleep in late, but get up early and get yourself moving.
- Avoid drinking caffeinated drinks such as cola, tea and coffee at bedtime. A herbal tea or a warm, milky drink is a better alternative.
- Sleep in a well-ventilated room, preferably with the window open.
- Avoid heavy meals late at night.
- Essential oils such as lavender, chamomile and marjoram all have sedative properties. Add a couple of drops of one of them to a warm bath before bedtime, or else put a couple of drops on to a paper tissue and place under the pillow.
- Hops can be dried and used to fill a "sleep cushion" for the bed. Alternatively, they can be brewed and made into a tea, to be drunk before you go to bed.

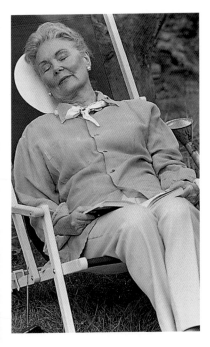

◂ If you can't sleep at night but find yourself falling asleep in the middle of the day, it's time to rethink your daily routine.

For animal lovers, keeping a pet can be **therapeutic**. If you feel a headache coming on, take the **dog** for a walk or sit and stroke your **cat** – you may find that the headache disappears.

# 12 laughter is the best medicine

Laughter is nature's tonic. It eases muscle tension, deepens breathing, improves circulation and releases headache-relieving endorphins to the brain to give you a natural "high".

If you feel you spend too much time working and not enough time having fun, or too much time on your own and not enough time with friends or family, try to redress the balance. Research shows there is a strong link between happiness and good health, so balance the stress of daily life by spending time regularly with friends and family.

▼ Laughter makes the world look brighter.

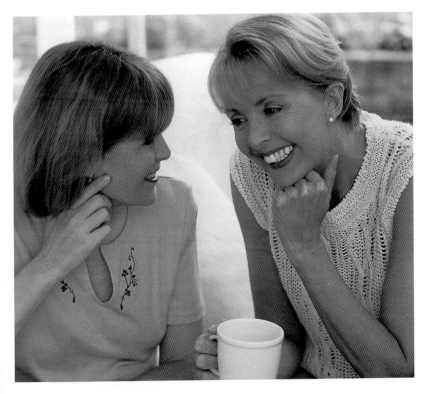

# 13 crystal healing

Crystals and stones magnify and transform energy, making them effective for healing purposes. There are many different crystals, but amethyst is very useful for soothing tension headaches.

**amethyst healing pattern**

This exercise focuses on freeing up the energy pathways between the neck and the head. You will need three or four washed amethyst points. Lie on your back on the floor in a warm place. Put one amethyst point on each side of the base of the neck, just above the collarbones, pointing up towards the top of the head. Place a third stone, pointing up, in the centre of the forehead on the brow chakra (third eye). A fourth amethyst can be placed, point outwards, at the top of the head, above the crown chakra. It is important to place the amethysts so that the points face upwards. This directs the flow of energy up through the neck and head and encourages the headache to lift.

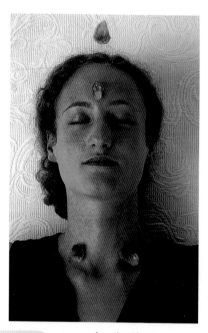

▲ Amethyst has a calming, protective quality and is helpful for mental disturbances. Its quietening effect makes it an excellent aid to meditation.

**CRYSTAL CLEANSING**

Because crystals act as energy transmitters, it is important to keep them clean. Before using them for healing they should always be washed in salt water. Ideally they should be left overnight, covered in salted water; the salt has a purifying action, helping to draw out any negativity which is being "held" in the stones. Always pour the water away.

# 14 headache healing spell

Try this ancient incantation to cure all types of headache. Before you make the spell, find a suitable tree to bury it under – ash, birch, juniper, orange and cedar trees all have healing powers.

**you will need**
gold candle and match
gold pen
15cm (6in) square of natural paper
knife
lime
gold cord
15cm (6in) square of orange cloth
spade

**1** Light the candle and invite your guardian angel or spirit helper to support the healing. Make up your own words, or say the following:

*I light this flame to honour
your presence and ask you to
hear this prayer.*

**2** Write your name clearly with the pen on the paper, at the same time visualizing a protective bubble of health and wellbeing surrounding you. Keep yourself focused.
**3** Cut the lime lengthways into two. Fold the paper three times and place it between the two lime halves. Bind the lime halves together with gold cord, while saying the following invocation (prayer):

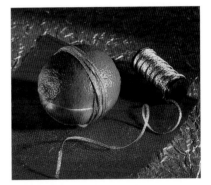

*Powers of lime,
Health is mine,
Cleanse the body,
Cleanse the mind,
Spirit pure,
Fill my being with health,
With health,
With health.*

**4** Place the bound lime in the orange cloth and bind the cloth with gold cord. Blow out the candle and say farewell to your higher self, guardian angel or spirit helper.
**5** Bury the parcel in the earth under your chosen tree. Ask the tree to help you return to good health and thank the tree.

# 15

# blue colour therapy

Colours can affect our mood and we can tap into this power to use colour for healing purposes. Blue is one of the best colours for calming and soothing frayed nerves.

To ease a tension headache, look for colours which have a calming and cooling effect on the mind and emotions. When you need rest and healing, blue is a good colour to choose. Blue is the colour of the seas and skies and is associated with peace and tranquillity. Soft and soothing blue is a perfect antidote to the stresses, strains and tensions of modern living.

You can work with colour in a variety of ways. The clothes you wear, the decor of your room and your personal possessions are some of the most obvious ways to bring colour into your life.

## changing the environment

Bathe yourself in coloured light using coloured films in combination with a free-standing spotlight. To do this, place a sheet of coloured film over the light, making sure that it is not touching the hot bulb. Turn off all the other lights and turn on the spotlight. If it is daytime, draw the curtains or blinds. Sit in the path of the spotlight's ray and bathe in the coloured light for an instant, on-the-spot therapy.

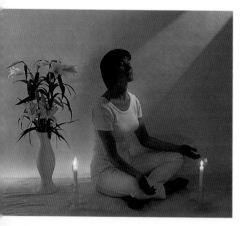

### COLOUR CHOICES

You may have noticed that your preference for particular colours varies over time. Start paying attention to which colours attract and which ones repel you. It may mean that you need more of the ones you are attracted to, and a bit less of the others.

◀ Blue is restful on the eye and is excellent for slowing things down.

# 16 green colour therapy

In the spectrum of colours, green lies centrally between red and blue. Green can have a balancing, harmonizing effect. The green of the natural world is nourishing to the spirits.

Take a walk in a leafy green forest and feel the colour green refresh and revitalize you. A walk in the country, taking in fresh air, has the same effect. For headaches arising from nervous exhaustion and debility, green is a good colour to work with. Green is the colour of harmony; it is an excellent tonic for the nerves and helps to restore stability when you are out of balance. Green is all around us in so many tonal values. Light, vibrant green in particular has an uplifting effect on the spirit and is useful when you are feeling depressed.

## colour vibration

One way of treating yourself is to have a selection of coloured silks which you can use to wrap yourself in. By wrapping coloured silk around your body, you envelop yourself in pure colour vibration. Choose the colour to which you feel most attracted for your treatment. Turquoise has a soothing and calming effect on the central nervous system.

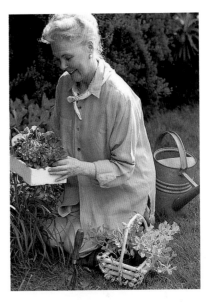

▲ When you are feeling drained, spend some time in a quiet park, garden or green fields and notice the effect on your energy levels.

**STRESS BUSTER**
If you don't have a large piece of cloth, a small, green silk square placed behind your head in a chair can relieve tension and pressure.

# 17 relax your body

Relaxation is as important for your health and wellbeing as exercise and a nutritious diet. If you do not switch off from the tensions of everyday life, you are more likely to suffer frequent headaches.

Breathing is something you do unconsciously, but when you are relaxed and calm your breathing pattern is different from when you are tense, anxious or negative. At times of great tension and stress, breathing is usually irregular and shallow, and does not completely fulfil your need for oxygen. If you learn to control your breathing it will help you to stay relaxed even in the most tense or stressful situations.

### breathe deeply

Working with the breath is one of the best ways to relax both mind and body. This technique is often used at the end of yoga or exercise sessions. Here is a simple breath control strategy that you can practise at any time. Learning to focus your attention on just your breathing and nothing else will enhance your body awareness and control and help to make you feel calm and centred.

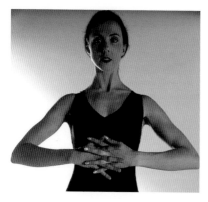

**1** Place your hands with your palms under your chest, on your ribs, and your fingers loosely interlocked. Inhale slowly and continuously through your nose, to a count of four. Do not strain, keep yourself relaxed.

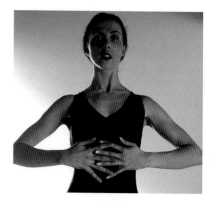

**2** As you inhale, concentrate on allowing your ribs to expand laterally: your fingers should gently part. Don't let your ribs jut forward. Exhale slowly, expelling all the breath from the lungs, then repeat.

# 18

# relax your mind

A short meditation break in the day will help your mind to unwind and help you return to your activities with a clear head. Meditating at night will help you to relax and prepare for sleep.

**visualization exercise**

Sit down in a comfortable spot where you won't be disturbed. Close your eyes and allow your mind to drift to a pleasant, peaceful place. A special place where you can relax… completely. A safe… secure… place … where nothing can ever bother you. It may be a place that you know … or one that you imagine. Perhaps a garden… or a place in the countryside … or maybe a room. But it is a place where you feel safe and able to let go… completely… a place that is unique and special to you.

When you are in your place… notice the light: is it bright, natural or dim? Notice also the temperature level… hot, warm or cool? Be aware of the colours that surround you… the shapes… and textures… the familiar objects that make that place special.

Continue to relax in your special place… enjoying the sounds… the smells… the atmosphere… with nobody wanting anything from you … just you in your special place where you can truly relax.

To end the meditation, slowly

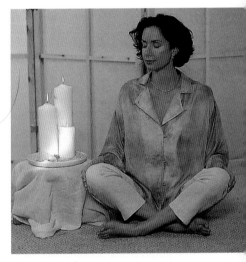

▲ Candlelit rooms help create the right mood for meditation.

bring your attention back to the room. When you are ready, open your eyes.

**CHANGE YOUR BRAINWAVES**
Meditation is one of the best forms of relaxation there is; in meditation, the brain-wave pattern changes to relaxed alpha waves, similar to the pattern shown in sleep.

# 19

## protective bubble visualization

Tap into the creative power of your imagination to increase your health and wellbeing and help remove the stress that causes headaches. Creative visualization is simple to learn and effective.

A lot of the stress of daily living comes from trying to satisfy the needs, demands and expectations of others. When the pressure becomes too much, it is easy to react by snapping angrily or by swallowing feelings of resentment and hostility. This is a classic scenario for a thumping headache. To protect yourself from outside pressure, try this visualization which involves creating a protective bubble or shield around yourself.

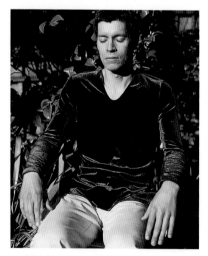

▲ *"Thinking yourself well" has many beneficial effects.*

### calm and clarity

Sit comfortably, close your eyes and imagine yourself in the kind of stressful situation that typically leads to a headache. Picture yourself and any other people who may be involved. Now notice a slight shimmer of light between yourself and the other people … a protective bubble around you. Learn to believe that this bubble only allows positive and helpful energies to reach you and reflects any negativity back to its source… leaving you free to get on with your life feeling calm and inwardly strong.

While you are in your bubble of light, imagine talking to someone who has been causing pressure to build. See yourself communicating with that person in a calm and clear way until they understand the position. Next, find unhelpful emotions such as past resentments and hurts and imagine pushing them out through the bubble where they can no longer limit or harm you. As you finish the visualization, remind yourself that the bubble stays with you, protecting you. Use this technique next time you feel a headache coming on.

# 20 gentle candlelight

Practically all headaches feel worse if you are surrounded by harsh bright light. The warm soft glow of candlelight creates a comforting and soothing ambience. Use it to help you unwind.

## choosing candles

To help a headache, combine some aroma and colour therapy and choose candles with healing scents and hues. Simple white candles are effective, or look for pale, soft colours, such as pinks and mauves which have a healing effect on the emotions. Avoid large candles in shades of vibrant red and orange, acid green and yellow or dark purple and black.

## soothing aromas

Scent is largely a matter of personal preference, but when you have a headache sickly sweet smells such as vanilla or heavy scents such as musk are probably best avoided. Some people like light floral scents, while others may prefer hints of fresh citrus. Sandalwood is also a good choice; this fragrance is traditionally used as a therapeutic aid to meditation, as it helps the mind to relax. Frankincense is another scent which is used in meditation; it has a calming effect on the nerves and slows down the breathing. If you don't like perfumed candles but would like to use scent, you could burn incense sticks or vaporize essential oils instead.

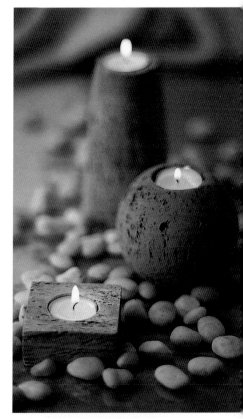

▲ A warm and uncluttered room is a good place to relax by candlelight. Make sure that the candles are in a suitable container to protect your furniture from hot candle wax.

# 21 clear the clutter

Too much paraphernalia in our lives makes us overburdened, depleting our energy and leaving us open to illness of all kinds. Keeping your space clutter-free keeps the energy pathways clear.

Books, papers and toys left lying around, untidy cupboards or work-spaces, anything that's kept "just in case", and any unfinished tasks or jobs which need to be done are all examples of clutter. When you start to accumulate junk, it's a fact that you will always add to it. Having piles of debris lying around, and items wrongly filed or waiting to be put away, will eventually wear you down and hinder your movement around a room. Once a whole house becomes cluttered, the effect is debilitating and depressing, leading to illness. Notice the effect on your energy levels after you have had a good clear-out.

**TASK LIST**
Make a list of all the jobs that need doing and put them in order of priority; make a point of tackling something on your list each day.

• Go through your cupboards and have a clear out at least twice a year. Throw out anything that you are not using and no longer need.
• Don't forget to clear places like the loft, garden shed and cellar. They are typical dumping grounds for clutter.
• Always keep your desk and work area clear.
• Deal with correspondence quickly and don't let things lie in your in-tray for too long.
• If you find it difficult to throw things away, then ask a friend to help you. They won't have an emotional attachment to your things, and will be able to offer you a more objective opinion.

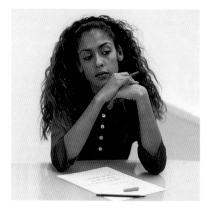

◀ *Make a list of any items you can sell, any jobs that need finishing or items that need mending, as you work through your space.*

# 22 healing homeopathy

Homeopathic remedies are prepared by diluting the original substance until what is left is a vibrational essence. These headache remedies stimulate the body to heal itself from within.

There are hundreds of remedies which are suitable for treating headaches, but below are some of the most widely available. Choose the remedy that most closely matches your symptoms. Take it three times a day in the 6C potency or once a day in the 30C potency until your symptoms have improved.

**Belladonna** for a throbbing, hammering headache that is worse at the temples, and the headache may be accompanied by fever.

**Euphrasia** for a headache accompanied by painful, watering eyes, where the sufferer is unable to bear bright light.

**Hypericum** for a pain that is lessened by bending the head backwards.

**Nat. Mur** for a migraine-type headache, which is preceded by misty vision or flickering lights in the eyes.

**Nux Vomica** to lessen the pain of a hangover headache.

**Pulsatilla** for a headache brought on by overwork, or associated with pre-menstrual tension or the menopause.

**Silica** for a headache that starts at the base of the neck and spreads up over the scalp, settling over the eyes.

**Sulphur** for a throbbing headache, which is improved when lying on the right and when gentle pressure is applied to the head.

▸ *Homeopathic remedies are made from plant, mineral and animal substances, some of which are highly poisonous in their original form. Because the remedies are diluted many times they are safe to use and have no harmful side effects.*

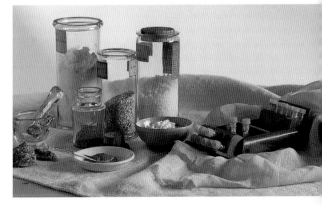

# 23 Reiki headache treatment

Reiki is a form of Japanese spiritual healing whereby chi, or "life energy", is channelled, in the case of a headache treatment, through the practitioner's hands on to the head of the sufferer.

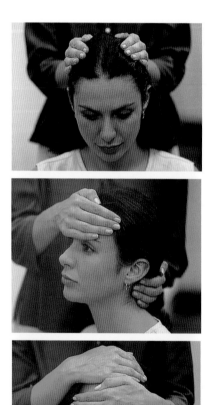

**1** Stand behind your partner and place both (warm) hands firmly on the sides of the head at the back, with your fingers coming up on to the top of the head. This cradling action feels very supportive and helps to dispel tension rising from the neck, balancing energy in the brain. Hold the position for a few minutes.

**2** Move to the side, and place one hand firmly on the forehead and the other at the base of the skull. Reiki works by putting the hands in certain positions on the body and then allowing the healing energy to flow through them. The aim of the treatment is to dissolve energy blocks and rebalance the body.

**3** Finish by placing one hand lightly over the eyes and the other on top of the head. This is very relaxing. After giving healing, you should always wash your hands. The person receiving reiki should drink plenty of water after the treatment to help flush out toxins. A reiki treatment can bring rapid relief to a headache.

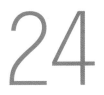

# 24 healing herb tub

Many of the remedies suggested in this book use plants. For quality and freshness, nothing beats growing your own. An attractive way of doing this is to plant up a container of healing herbs.

Use a large container to give the plants room to grow and site it in a sunny spot near the house for easy access.

**you will need**
Half-barrel
Bricks
Drainage material
Soilless compost (growing medium)
Sharp sand
Watering can

**plants**
Feverfew (*Tanacetum parthenium*)
Lavender (*Lavandula* 'Hidcote', *L.stoechas*)
Marjoram (*Origanum vulgare* 'Variegatum')
Rosemary (*Rosmarinus officinalis*), prostrate and upright forms
Lemon balm (*Melissa officinalis*)

1 Rest the tub on a few bricks to raise it off the ground and promote better drainage. Cover the base with a layer of drainage material such as broken pots, broken polystyrene plant trays or horticultural grit. Almost fill the tub with a 50/50 mixture of compost and sharp sand.

2 Arrange the herbs, still in their pots, on the surface of the compost. When you are happy with the arrangement, make holes and plant them, firming the compost down and topping up if necessary. Leave a gap below the rim of the tub to allow for watering. Water the plants in well.

▼ *Keep the plants well trimmed and replace the top layer of compost annually. Feed regularly in the summer months.*

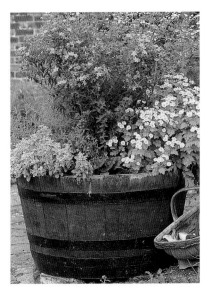

# 25

## gentle lavender & rosemary oils

There are many essential oils which can help treat a headache, but two of the most popular and effective are lavender and rosemary, which are both from the same plant family.

Lavender is particularly good for headaches that are related to stress and tension, while rosemary is useful for ones brought on by mental fatigue and nervous exhaustion; either is useful for headaches associated with depression. A quick and convenient headache treatment is to mix a drop of either oil in a teaspoon of carrier oil, such as almond. Rub the mix into your temples. Or put a drop of neat oil on a handkerchief and inhale the aroma.

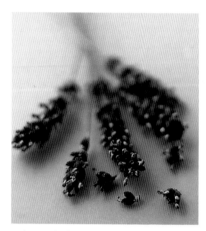

▲ Lavender has many healing properties. It is an excellent headache remedy as it is a natural analgesic.

▼ Rosemary helps to regulate blood pressure and can reduce pain.

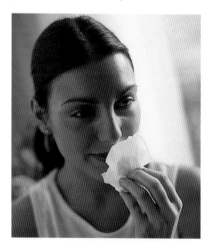

### HOW OILS WORK
Inhalation is the fastest way of enjoying the benefits of aromatic oils, as nerve pathways lead directly from the lining of the nose to the brain, having an immediate effect on the central nervous system.

**CAUTION:** Do not use rosemary oil if you are pregnant or suffer from epilepsy.

# 26 soothing bath water

Make up this bubble bath mix and keep it on standby for when you need to relax at the end of a long, stressful day – it will ease a headache and promote restful sleep.

## lavender bubble bath

The recipe uses dried lavender flowers as well as lavender oil for extra strength. The mixture will keep for several months in a cool, dark place.

### you will need

medium-sized bottle of clear, mild, unscented shampoo
45ml/3 tbsp dried lavender flowers
5 drops lavender essential oil
wide-necked, screw-topped glass jar
fine sieve
glass or plastic jug (pitcher)
squeezable plastic bottle

**1** Pour the shampoo, the lavender flowers and the lavender oil into the glass jar. Replace the lid and shake vigorously to mix all the ingredients thoroughly together.

**2** Leave this mixture to stand in a warm place, such as a sunny windowsill, for up to two weeks, shaking and turning the jar occasionally. The lavender flowers will infuse the shampoo.

**3** Strain off the lavender liquid into the jug and then pour it into the squeezable plastic bottle. Discard the dried lavender flowers.

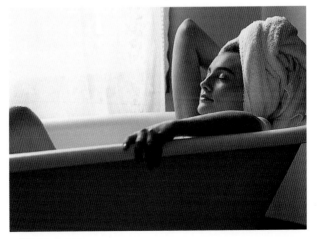

▸ *Let the day's tensions melt away with the delicate fragrance of lavender. Lavender is a recognized cure-all for many common ailments, including tense, nervous headaches.*

# 27

## a relaxing atmosphere

Scenting the environment can soothe a headache and help you regain equilibrium quickly. Try using a vaporizer with a few drops of your favourite essential oil.

The bedroom and bathroom are both ideal places to relax, while the use of soft music, candles and essential oil burners is a popular way of creating a peaceful and soothing atmosphere. Essential oil burners have a small dish to hold water and a source of gentle heat underneath, often a night-light candle. The heat needs to be fairly low, but warm enough to heat up the water. A few drops of essential oil are added to the warm water, which then slowly evaporates, giving out its scent. Alternatively, oil drops can be added to a bowl of hot water if you do not have a burner.

Any of the following oils will help to create a relaxing atmosphere. Add two or three drops to a burner.

**Clary Sage** for stress and tension headaches.

**Geranium** for headaches caused by premenstrual syndrome.

**Lavender** for migraine and tension headaches.

**Neroli** for headaches caused by mental exertion.

**Rose** to soothe and calm the nerves.

**Sweet Marjoram** for headaches caused by anxiety and insomnia.

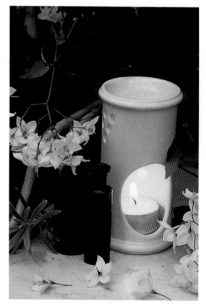

▲ Essential oils help speed up the healing process. Use them as an aid to recovery, as well as to scent your room.

**BE PREPARED**
Carry a small bottle of your favourite essential oil with you and try dabbing this on a handkerchief before reaching for the painkillers.

# 28 soothing away eyestrain

Many headaches are caused by eyestrain.
Watching a lot of television, working in poor light,
long-distance driving or sitting for long periods in
front of a computer screen can trigger headaches.

If your eyes are feeling tired and ache and you feel a headache coming on, you can give them a treat by covering them with cucumber slices. Or, if you are at work, you could try splashing cold water on to your eyes for a similar effect.

Alternatively, make eye-packs out of chamomile tea bags. Chamomile has a very gentle, anti-inflammatory, calming action. It helps alleviate sore, tired eyes and headaches arising from tension and anxiety. Boil a kettle and pour the hot water on to two tea bags. Leave to infuse for 10 minutes, then take them out of the water. Let them cool down and squeeze out any excess water. Lie back and place the bags over your eyes for a soothing effect.

**COMPUTER USERS**
If you use a computer, there are some simple steps you can take to reduce the likelihood of getting headaches from eyestrain:
• Take a short break away from your desk every 20–30 minutes.
• Make sure the computer has a good quality display and is fitted with an anti-glare filter. Adjust the brightness level on the screen to suit you.
• Set the computer screen at eye-level and position it so that it does not reflect glare from any other source of light, such as a window behind you, for instance.

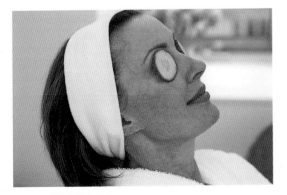

◄ Cucumber has a cooling, refreshing effect and helps to increase the circulation to the eye area.

# 29 feverfew

This bitter, edible plant has long been recognized as one of the most effective natural treatments for headaches and migraine. Feverfew works best as a prophylactic, taken over a period of time.

## migraine cure

Science attributes the action of feverfew to a natural chemical which seems to inhibit the release of the hormone serotonin, which is thought to be a migraine trigger. A three-month course of feverfew can reduce the number and severity of attacks.

Feverfew can be taken in tablet form. Check the label and make sure the pills contain at least 0.2 per cent of the active ingredient, parthenolide. A daily dose of 200mg is usually sufficient. Alternatively, many headache and migraine sufferers have been helped by eating the fresh leaves. Eat two to three leaves daily in a brown bread sandwich. The bread makes the bitter leaves more palatable. You may also use a little honey to sweeten them.

**CAUTION**
• Avoid feverfew during pregnancy and while breastfeeding.
• Too much fresh feverfew can cause side effects, including mouth ulcers, stomach pain and swollen lips.
• If you are taking other medication, discuss with your doctor first.

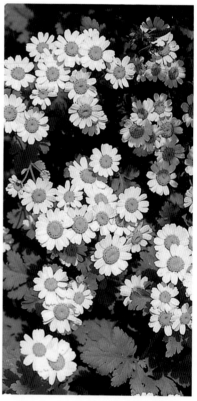

▲ Feverfew is easy to grow and can be used fresh or dried to treat headaches and migraine. The dried plant is also used to make feverfew tablets, available in good pharmacies and health stores.

# 30 evening primrose

For many women, headaches are a recognized symptom of PMS and of the menopause, and some women notice more headaches when taking the pill or hormone replacement therapy.

## hormonal regulator

Evening primrose is a traditional North American Indian medicine and enjoys a reputation as one of nature's most valuable and versatile remedies. A great deal of research has been done on the medicinal effect of the oil, which is extracted from the plants' seeds. It is a good source of Omega-6 fatty acids, vital for the healthy functioning of the immune, nervous and hormonal systems. In particular, the oil contains gamma-linoleic acid (GLA), which is especially helpful to counter hormonal problems.

Increasingly, many women regularly take a supplement of evening primrose oil, which is available in capsule form in pharmacies and health stores. The oil is not only helpful for treating PMS, but also migraine and menopausal problems. Medicinal doses range from 500–1500mg a day or as directed by a healthcare professional.

◄ The evening primrose plant has fragrant yellow cup-shaped flowers which open at dusk.

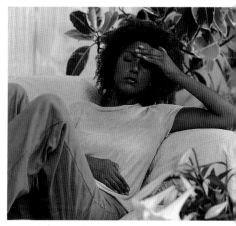

▲ Women who suffer from migraine are most likely to suffer attacks around the time of their periods.

### HANGOVER CURE
Evening primrose oil has also been shown to counter the effects of alcoholic poisoning. For a hangover headache, try taking a couple of capsules instead of a painkiller.

### CAUTION
Evening primrose should be avoided by women with breast cancer and sufferers of epilepsy.

# 31 herbal steam inhalant

A stuffy nose and blocked sinuses can sometimes be the cause of a headache. Steam inhalations are a good way of clearing the head. The addition of fresh herbs will help to relieve the headache.

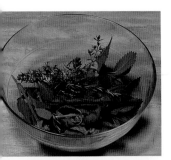

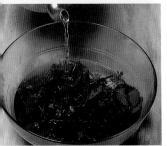

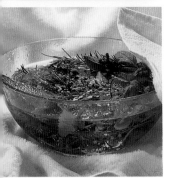

**1** To clear the sinuses and ease a congestive headache, gather together a large handful of lavender, rosemary, peppermint, sage, thyme and eucalyptus. Put the selected herbs in a bowl.

**2** Pour on 1 litre/ 1¾ pints/4 cups of boiling water. Lavender and rosemary are natural painkillers, while peppermint and eucalyptus are good for clearing blocked noses and throats.

**3** Lean over the bowl, with a towel draped over your head and shoulders to form a tent. Breathe in the steamy vapour as deeply as possible. The inhalation will decongest blocked nasal passages, kill any germs and clear the headache.

**TIPS**
• If fresh herbs are not available, then an inhalation using essential oils of peppermint, eucalyptus, lavender and rosemary may be tried instead. Use 2 drops of each oil to 1 litre/1¾ pints/4 cups of boiling water.

• The hormonal action of thyme can help lift depression and the symptoms of fatigue.

**CAUTION**
If you have high blood pressure or asthma, seek medical advice before using steam inhalants. Eucalyptus and peppermint may interfere with homeopathic remedies.

# 32

# comforting compress

Many headache sufferers find a compress helps their symptoms. A compress is a cloth which has been soaked in water with a few drops of essential oil added, wrung out, then applied to the head.

Of all the essential oils used in the treatment of headaches, lavender and peppermint seem to be the most effective. Although they can be used separately, these oils work well together. Both are painkillers and complement each other: lavender is a sedative while peppermint is a stimulant. This dual action is found in many commercial headache remedies, which include a stimulant (such as caffeine) to counteract the slightly sedative, and even depressing effect of the painkiller. The important difference is that essential oils do not just suppress the pain but get to work on the cause of the headache. A compress will be most effective if it is used immediately at the onset of a headache.

**you will need**
600ml/1 pint/2½ cups cold water
bowl
2–3 drops lavender essential oil
2–3 drops peppermint essential oil
piece of soft cotton fabric

**1** Pour the water into the bowl. When the water is still add the essential oils and gently stir the water to disperse the oils.
**2** Fold the soft cotton fabric into a loose pad. Place it on the surface of the water and let it soak up the essential oils. Wring it out lightly.
**3** Place the compress across the forehead to relieve the headache. As soon as it gets warm, soak it again in the water and re-apply.

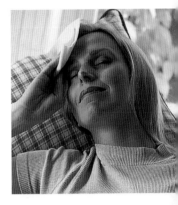

**TIPS**
• During a migraine attack, some sufferers cannot tolerate the smell of peppermint, in which case try alternating hot and cold lavender compresses.
• A cold compress on the back of the neck will ease a tension headache, and one on the forehead is best for a thumping headache.

# 33

## lime blossom & lemon balm tisane

A simple but effective way of curing a headache is to drink a herbal tea. Lime blossom and lemon balm (*Melissa*) leaves make a delicately fragranced drink for soothing tension headaches.

### herbal infusions

Making herbal tisanes from fresh ingredients increases their potency and medicinal value. Lime flowers have a relaxing and cleansing effect in the body. They can help with high blood pressure, and are effective in treating headaches, including migraine. Lime flowers make a good remedy for any condition associated with tension, including depression, and back, neck and shoulder pain. Lemon balm is useful for calming tension and promoting feelings of wellbeing; it can also relieve headaches and migraine. The two herbs are complementary.

To make this tisane, gather a handful each of lemon balm leaves and lime blossom – pick lime blossom when the flowers are just opening. Use five or six fresh flowers and leaves per cup, and drop them into near-boiling water. Cover and leave to steep for three or four minutes. Strain off the liquid and drink hot or cold, three times a day. The tea has a fresh, lemony taste.

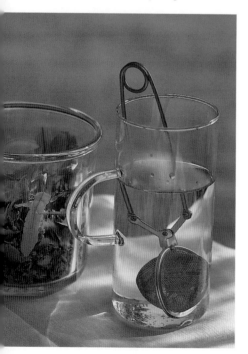

◀ *Lime blossom can also be mixed with peppermint for a more uplifting effect.*

**CAUTION**
Although natural, herbal teas can be potent and should be taken no more than three times a day and for no more than two weeks at a time.

# wood betony infusion

Once considered a panacea for all ills, wood
betony may be used alone or combined
with lavender or rosemary to make a soothing
herbal infusion to ease your headache.

The leaves and pink flowering tops of
wood betony are used in medicinal
preparations. The plant has a stimulating
effect on the circulation and is also a
relaxant, making it helpful for both
congestive and tension headaches. It is
also a tonic to the nervous system,
helping to ease anxiety, lift depression
and soothe pain.

The infusion may be made with
either fresh or dried ingredients. Fill
a cup with near-boiling water and
add 5ml/1 tsp dried wood betony
and 2.5ml/½ tsp dried lavender or
rosemary. Double these quantities if
you are using fresh herbs. Cover and
leave to steep for 10 minutes. Strain
and drink, sweetened with a little
honey if required.

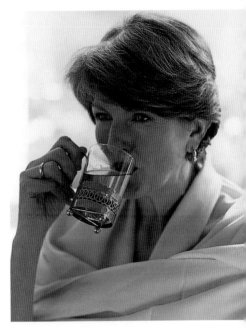

▲ Wood betony was highly prized as a
medicinal herb in Roman times. The
Anglo-Saxons believed it capable of driving
away despair.

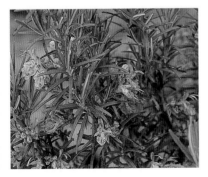

◀ Fresh rosemary is invigorating and
refreshing. It is excellent for clearing
congestive headaches, and combines
well with wood betony to relieve
nervous tension.

**nature's medicine chest / 45**

# 35 herbal sedatives

Headaches caused by stress and nervous exhaustion are generally linked with an inability to switch the mind off and relax, leading to insomnia and restless nights.

## calming the nerves

There are several herbs which have a strong sedative action and which are useful for headaches associated with nervous exhaustion and overactivity. Among the most commonly used are valerian, vervain and sweet marjoram: any one of these can be made into an infusion that will help you to relax and promote restful, healing sleep. Do not take all three together.

For every 250ml/8fl oz/1 cup of near-boiling water you will need 10ml/2 tsp of fresh valerian, vervain or sweet marjoram. If using dried herbs, halve the quantity. Drop the herbs into the water, cover and leave to infuse for 5–10 minutes. Strain off the liquid, sweeten with a little honey, and drink before going to bed.

> **CAUTION**
> Sweet marjoram and vervain should not be taken during pregnancy. Valerian should not be taken by anyone with liver disease.

▲ Vervain is a wonderful tonic for the nervous system, calming the nerves and easing tension. It protects against stress, and is useful for treating headaches caused by anxiety, depression and insomnia.

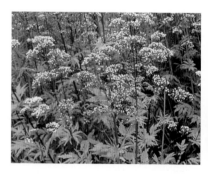

▲ Valerian has a calming effect on the mind and helps to relax tense muscles – use it to ease a tight neck and shoulders. It is a strong sedative, and forms the basis of the pharmaceutical drug, valium.

# 36 lavender tincture

Tinctures are an effective way to extract the active ingredients of plants. They are made with fresh or dried herbs which are steeped in a mixture of alcohol and water. This one will cure a headache.

**you will need**
15g/½oz dried lavender
250ml/8fl oz/1 cup vodka, made
  up to 300ml/½ pint/1¼ cups
  with water
dark glass jar with an airtight lid

**1** Put the dried lavender into a glass jar and pour in the vodka and water mixture. It will almost immediately start to turn a beautiful lavender blue.
**2** Put a lid on the jar and leave in a cool, dark place for 7–10 days (no longer), shaking the jar occasionally. The tincture will eventually turn dark purple.
**3** Strain off the lavender through a sieve lined with a paper towel before pouring into a sterilized glass bottle. Seal with a tight-fitting lid and store in a cool, dark place for future use.

As tinctures are highly concentrated medicinal extracts, take no more than 5ml/1 tsp, three or four times a day, as a headache treatment. The tincture may be diluted in a little water or fruit juice. Alternatively, a few drops may be added to a compress.

**MEDICINE CHEST**
• Among herbal remedies, tinctures have a relatively long shelf-life; properly stored, they will keep for up to two years, as the alcohol acts as a preservative.
• Lavender tincture is a useful remedy to have on standby as it can be used to treat many common health problems, such as burns, muscular aches and pains, coughs and colds, as well as headaches of all kinds.

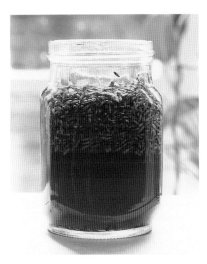

# 37

## hangover headache treatments

Waking up with a hangover takes all the fun out of the night before. Before dashing off for the black coffee, try some natural remedies. There are many simple things you can do which are effective.

**fruit sugar**

Hangover headaches seem to result from metabolic disturbances in the brain as a result of drinking too much alcohol. Experts think this may cause a type of "brain hypoglycemia" or low blood sugar, which is why some people recommend eating a snack before going to bed that is high in fructose (fruit sugar). Research suggests that fructose helps metabolize the chemical products of alcohol that cause headaches and hangovers. Fructose is found in carrots, and in all fruits, especially dates. Fructose bars are also available in health stores.

**rehydrate**

It's important to drink plenty of water and to increase your intake of vitamin C. Alcohol dehydrates the body; drinking water counters this effect, and helps to flush out toxins. Vitamin C is needed for more than 300 metabolic processes in the body.

Kiwi fruit and all citrus fruits are a good natural source. Make a drink from freshly squeezed orange or lemon juice, sweeten it with honey and it will help the headache.

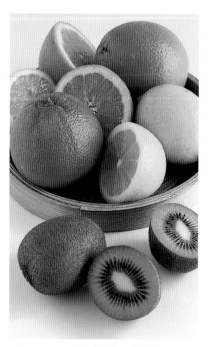

▲ *Oranges and kiwi fruit are high in vitamin C.*

You could also keep a supply of homeopathic nux vomica at home. Sometimes, a single dose is enough to clear up nausea and a thumping headache. Take it in a 6C potency every hour for up to eight doses.

# 38

# Bach flower remedies

The Bach flower remedies work on any underlying emotional or psychological cause of a headache, treating the negative mental and emotional states which lead to pain and tension in the body.

Dr Edward Bach discovered the healing energies of selected flowering plants and trees, by "tuning in" to their subtle vibrations. He noted that the plants affected him on a mental and emotional level, and devised a system of healing based on these states. The remedies match certain personality types and are chosen accordingly.

Bach flower essences are gentle and safe to use and are available in most pharmacies and health stores. They may be taken separately or in a combination of up to six remedies. They may also be taken in conjunction with other treatments. Add a couple of drops of each essence to a glass of water and sip at frequent intervals.

## FLOWER ESSENCES
To treat a headache, select from the following remedies:
- **Beech** if you are critical and intolerant of others and yourself.
- **Cherry Plum** if you have repressed anger and feel as if you might explode, or feel fearful.
- **Crab Apple** if you try to be "superman/woman", or are driven by the need to be perfect.
- **Gorse** if you have feelings of hopelessness and are resigned to fate.
- **Holly** if you suffer from feelings of jealousy, hatred, resentment and frustration.
- **Impatiens** if you feel tension due to rapid mental activity, or are always in a hurry.
- **Pine** if you have feelings of guilt and inferiority, if you always blame yourself or are always apologizing.
- **Vervain** if you live on your nerves, are keyed up and unable to relax.
- **Vine** if you are rigid in your thinking, if you are inflexible or ambitious, or if you think you are always right.
- **White Chestnut** for thoughts that go round and round.

▲ There are 38 Bach essences.

# 39 calming head massage

Gentle massage of the temples and forehead can help to stop a tension headache from getting a tight grip and encourage the body to relax. Use essential oils for additional benefit.

Everyone can benefit from the comforting touch of massage. The sense of touch is a powerful tool of communication and can be used to benefit the recipient on an emotional, physical and mental level. It helps relaxation, relieves aching muscles and reduces pain making it a useful treatment for headaches.

Add any of the essential oils in the quantity stated in the box, right, to 30ml/2 tbsp of a light vegetable oil, such as almond or grapeseed, or to an unscented cream or lotion.

**CHOOSING AN OIL**
• **Rosemary** for a congestive headache. Rosemary is uplifting and clears the mind. Use 4 drops.
• **Peppermint** if the head feels too hot (peppermint has a cooling action). Use 4 drops.
• **Lavender** if warmth feels as though it is helpful. Use 6 drops.
• **Chamomile** for either headaches or migraine. Use 4 drops.
• **Marjoram** when the mind simply won't switch off. Use 4 drops.

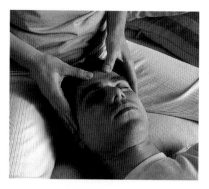

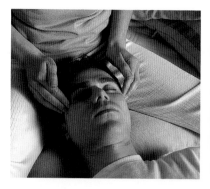

1 With your thumbs, use steady but gentle pressure to stroke the forehead and work the oils into the skin. The strokes will help ease tension.

2 Gently massage the temples with the tips of your fingers to release tension and stress. Work the oils into the skin as before.

# 40 neck & shoulder easer

Sitting hunched over a desk for long periods, driving, or carrying heavy bags are just a few of the occupational hazards that create tension in the shoulders, neck and below the ridge of the skull.

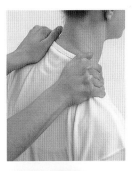

**1** Anchor your fingers over the shoulders. Roll and squeeze the muscles in a kneading action, working out to the edge of the shoulders and down the tops of the arms.

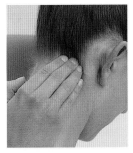

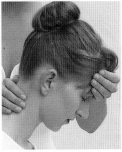

**2** Place one hand across the forehead and the other across the nape of the neck. Squeeze the neck muscles between the fingers and heel of your hand.

**4** Loosen the constricted muscles under the base of the skull by massaging beneath the bony ridge, working from the top of the spine to the outer edge of the skull.

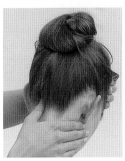

**3** Supporting the forehead, use the thumb pad of the other hand to press upwards into the hollow at the top of the spine below the skull. Apply gentle upward pressure for a steady count of five, then release.

**5** Change hands to massage beneath the other side of the skull. Ease scalp tension by rotating the fingertips of both hands in small circles all over the head.

# 41

# shoulder reliever

Having a shoulder massage is one of the best ways of releasing muscular tension. It not only feels good, but can help to prevent or ease a headache. Practise this routine with a friend or your partner.

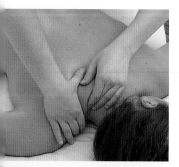

**1** Make sure your partner faces away from you. Place both your hands on one shoulder, and with alternate hands squeeze your fingers and thumb together. Repeat on the other side.

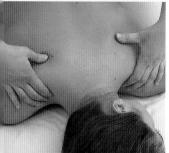

**2** Place your thumbs on each side of the spine on the upper back, with the rest of each hand over each shoulder. Squeeze your fingers and thumbs together, rolling the flesh between them.

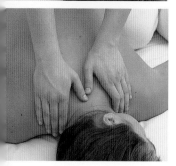

**3** Let your thumbs smoothly move out across the shoulder muscles, and release the pressure of the thumbs as you stretch the shoulder blades outwards, away from the spine, with your hands.

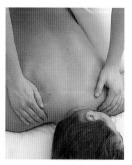

**4** Return your hands to the centre and repeat this movement with a firm kneading action.

**RELAX**
A typical response to feeling burdened by life's responsibilities is to tighten up in the trapezius, the large muscle in the shoulders. We hold a lot of tension in this area; when you feel "uptight" it is often the shoulders that bear the load. Make a conscious effort to relax your shoulders.

# 42 anxiety calmer

When you are feeling anxious and upset, the
muscles of the face tense up, making you look
fraught. Having the face gently massaged is very
relaxing, and a great way to soothe a headache.

Ask a friend to practise this routine with you. It is best done when you have an opportunity to relax afterwards. For a headache, it is a good idea to use essential oils, blended in a little massage oil. Choose a light vegetable oil, such as sweet almond or grapeseed, as a base. Use four or five drops of essential oil to 30ml/ 2 tbsp massage oil, but take care not to put too much on at a time, as most people don't like a greasy feeling on the face. If you prefer, you may use an unscented lotion or cream as a base.

1 Ideally have the person lying down with the head on a cushion. With your fingertips, smooth the essential oil blend into the face. Pay particular attention to the temples and forehead, using small circular movements and light brushing strokes.

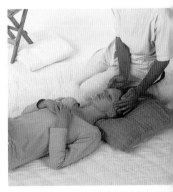

2 Using your thumbs one after the other, stroke tension away from the centre of the forehead. Finish the routine by holding your hands still on each side of the face; this feels very calming and reassuring.

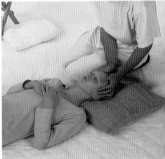

**ESSENTIAL OILS**
• **Chamomile** or **marjoram** for headaches that are the result of overwork, anger or worry.
• **Lavender** for migraine and tension headaches.
• **Tea tree** for clearing the head.

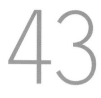

# Shiatsu massage

This traditional Japanese healing system is based on applying pressure to the body, and using stretching and holding movements. This routine is excellent in the treatment of tension headaches.

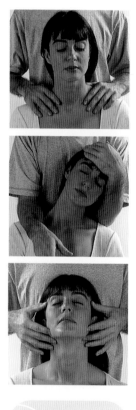

**1** Standing behind your partner, place both hands loosely on each side of the neck. Gently massage the shoulders to help relax the breathing.

**2** Tilt the head sideways and support with your hand. Place the forearm across the shoulder and apply downward pressure. Repeat on the other side.

**3** Apply gentle pressure with the thumb and forefinger from the base of the neck to the nape. Hold at the nape for 5 seconds, then release. Tilt the head back, supporting it. Place your thumbs on the temples with the fingers resting on each side of the face. Rotate the thumbs in small forward movements.

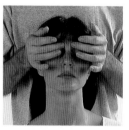

**4** Find the pressure points just above the inner corner of each eye. Apply gentle pressure with the middle fingers to help disperse the pain. Hold for 5 seconds.

**5** Position your thumbs about 5cm/2in apart on each side of the head, just above the hairline, with the palms pressed flat along the sides of the face. Press the thumbs evenly back along the top of the head.

**POSTURE**
Sit on an upright chair with good back support.

# 44

## foot reflexology

The science of reflexology believes that our bodies are reflected in miniature in our feet. If we treat the specific area of the foot that represents the head, we can massage away a headache.

**an ancient art**

Having a reflexology treatment is relaxing and can treat specific health problems. It is effective for treating tension headaches as well as for migraines.

Your head is represented on the toes; the right side of your head lies on the right big toe and the left side on the left big toe. In addition, the eight other toes contain the reflexes to specific parts of your head, for fine tuning. By applying gentle pressure to these exact points, reflexology stimulates the body to heal itself.

Reflexology can be an excellent preventive therapy. If the headache is a symptom of another illness, a different part of the foot to that suggested here would need to be treated first.

**1** Work the hypothalmus reflex first, as this controls the release of endorphins for the relief of pain.

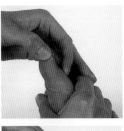

**2** Work down the spine to take pressure away from the head. This will draw energy down the body and ground it.

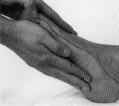

**3** Work the cervical spine on the big toe. Work the neck of all the toes to relieve tension.

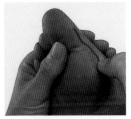

**4** Work the diaphragm to encourage freer breathing. Repeat the reflexology treatment on the other foot.

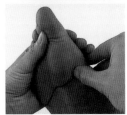

# 45 scalp massage

A scalp massage is deeply relaxing. If you are suffering from stress-related headaches, use this treatment on a regular basis to reduce tension. It only takes a few minutes.

If you are stressed, the scalp muscles tighten. One side effect is that the roots of your hair become starved of nourishment and your hair will start to thin out and weaken. This massage stimulates the hair roots. The advantage of this massage is that it is one you can do for yourself.

▸ *Lank, lifeless hair may be an early sign of stress.*

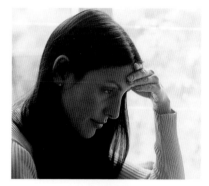

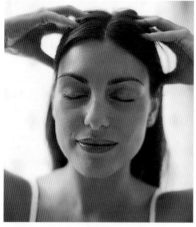

**1** Place the thumbs at the top of the ears and "glue" the fingers to the scalp, moving it firmly and slowly over the bone beneath.

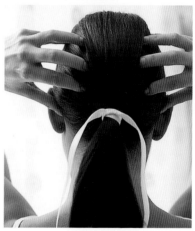

**2** Place the hands on another part of the scalp and repeat. Carry on until the whole scalp has been covered. Repeat steps 1 and 2 several times.

# 46 head revitalizer

This simple self-massage sequence will help to ease headaches, whatever their cause. You can also use it to increase your vitality and help you to focus your mind throughout the day.

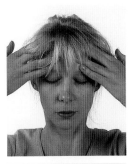

1 Use small, circling movements with the fingers, working steadily from the forehead down around the temples and over the cheeks.

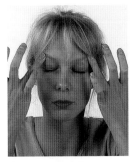

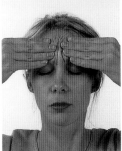

2 Use firm pressure and work slowly to ease tensions out of all the facial muscles. Use your fingers to gently press around the eye sockets, by the nose.

4 Try not to pull downwards on the skin – let the circling movements help to smooth the stresses away and gently lift the face as you work.

**USE AN OIL**
If you are feeling overwrought, make up an aromatherapy blend of 4 drops lavender and 2 drops ylang ylang in 30ml/ 2 tbsp of a light massage oil, such as sweet almond or grapeseed.

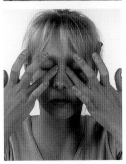

3 Smooth firmly around the arcs of the eye sockets. Work across the cheeks and along each side of the nose, then move out to the jaw line where a lot of tension is held.

# 47 migraine easers

Having a migraine is one of nature's ways of shutting the body down when things get too much. Rather than trying to "fight it off", respect what your body is saying and look after yourself.

There are several essential oils which can help a migraine, but use them sparingly and carefully. Many migraine sufferers have a heightened sense of smell at the onset of an attack, and may find any aroma intolerable.

**massage mix**
As soon as you feel a migraine coming on, try a massage blend of 2 drops rosemary, 1 drop marjoram, and 1 drop clary sage oil, diluted in 30ml/2 tbsp of a light vegetable oil, such as grapeseed or sweet almond. You may use an unscented lotion or cream base rather than oil if you prefer.

Alternatively, use a drop of each oil in a bowl of warm water, and apply a warm compress to the forehead. If this blend smells too strong, you could just try lavender on its own, 3–4 drops in the base oil or cream as before.

**1** Using the massage mix, gently rub the temples with small circular movements, using the tips of your fingers.
**2** If touching the head does not make the pain worse, ask a friend to give you a gentle head massage. This can feel very soothing and comforting and help you to relax.

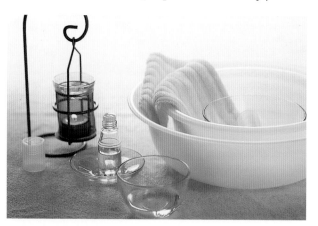

◄ *Migraine headaches are not the same as everyday tension headaches, and if you suffer from these you should seek professional advice.*

# 48 calming sleep massage

The gentle wave-like strokes of this massage wash over and down the body with a deliciously hypnotic and sedative effect – ideal to ease away headaches before going to sleep.

**1** Place one hand over the chest and the other over the back of the shoulder. As you breathe in, pull your hands steadily outwards and down to the edge of the shoulder. Pause briefly as you exhale, lightly cradling the top of the arm.

**2** Continue the pulling motion down the length of the arm. As you breathe in, pull both hands down to just below the elbow joint. Relax as you breathe out, then continue the slide down the forearm and below the wrist.

**3** Draw your hands over both sides of your partner's hand and fingers, taking your stroke out beyond the body as the hand settles back on to the mattress. Repeat steps 1–3 on the other side of the body.

**4** Pull your hands down over the hips and down the leg to just below the knee. Continue this wave-like motion down the lower leg to the ankle, then pull gently and steadily out over the toes. Repeat this sequence of strokes on the other side of the body. Repeat each movement up to five times.

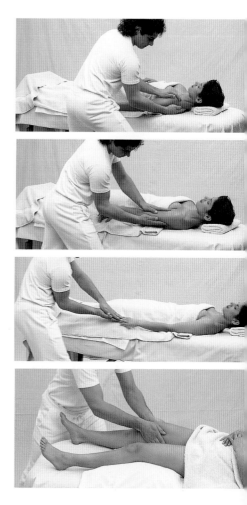

# 49 draw out the pain

Certain techniques can help to release the pain of a tension headache. Those shown here all involve applying pressure then releasing it. This helps to relax the muscles and draw the pain away.

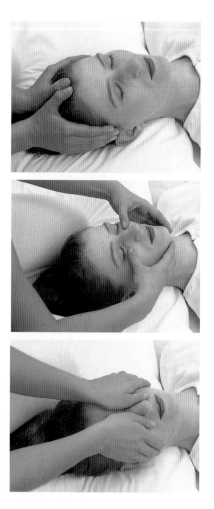

**1** Settle your hands lightly around your partner's scalp for a few moments. Keeping your hands in the cupped position, lift them slowly away from the head as if they are drawing out the pain. Cup your hands around the head again, placing your thumbs between the eyebrows. Apply gentle pressure with your thumbs for a count of five, then release.

**2** Working from inner to outer edge, apply a press/release motion under the ridge of both eyebrows using the tips of your index fingers. Then use your thumb pads to press/release over the top of the cheekbones, working out from the nose to the edge of the temples.

**3** Briskly rub your hands together to create heat, then softly lay your slightly cupped palms over the eyes for a count of five to soothe and relax the eye muscles. Withdraw your hands slowly.

# 50 tension reliever

Tension headaches are a common consequence of stressful lifestyles. This massage can prevent muscle spasm and head pain, particularly if it is done at the onset of a headache.

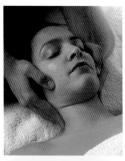

1 Kneel at your partner's head with the head in your lap or on a cushion. Begin by making circles with your fingertips on the muscles at each side of the neck. Continue around the sides of the head and behind the ears.

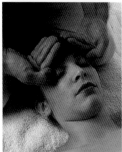

2 Use the backs of your hands to smooth tension away from the temples. Gently stroke the hands outwards across the forehead to soothe away worry lines.

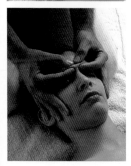

3 Pinch and gently squeeze along the line of the eyebrows, reducing pressure as you work outwards. These muscles may be very tender, so take care.

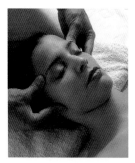

4 With your thumbs, use steady but firm pressure on the forehead, working outwards from between the eyebrows.

5 Work across the brow to the hair line. This also covers many acupressure points, and will release blocked energy.

# index

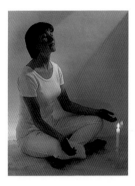
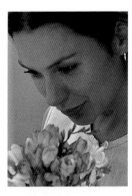

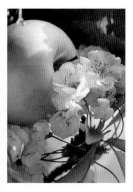
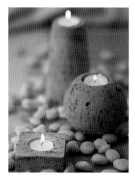

This edition is published by Lorenz Books,
an imprint of Anness Publishing Ltd,
Blaby Road, Wigston, Leicestershire LE18 4SE; info@anness.com

www.lorenzbooks.com; www.annesspublishing.com

If you like the images in this book and would like to investigate using them
for publishing, promotions or advertising, please visit our website
www.practicalpictures.com for more information.

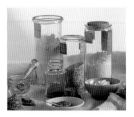

A CIP catalogue record for this book is available from the
British Library.

Publisher: Joanna Lorenz
Managing Editor: Helen Sudell
Editor: Simona Hill
Designer: Lisa Tai
Production Controller: Helen Wang
Photographers: Sue Atkinson, Michelle Garrett, Christine
Hanscomb, Janine Hosegood, Alistair Hughs, Andrea Jones, Don
Last, Liz McAulay and Debbie Patterson

**Publisher's note:**
The reader should not regard the recommendations, ideas and techniques
expressed and described in this book as substitutes for the advice of a qualified
medical practitioner or other qualified professional. Any use to which
the recommendations, ideas and techniques are put is at the reader's
sole discretion and risk.

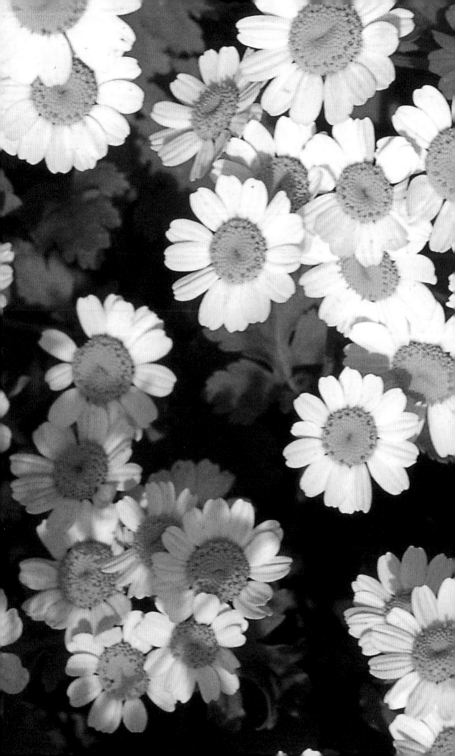